Sugar Detox Cookbook

The 21 Day Cookbook for Rapid Weight Loss, Unstoppable Energy, Intense Focus, and an End to Sugar Cravings – Over 45 Recipes

Michelle Jones

hardship or damages that may befall them after undertaking information described herein.

Additionally, the information found on the following pages is intended for informational purposes only and should thus be considered, universal. As befitting its nature, the information presented is without assurance regarding its continued validity or interim quality. Trademarks that are mentioned are done without written consent and can in no way be considered an endorsement from the trademark holder.

Table of Contents

Introduction

Congratulations on downloading this book and thank you for doing so.

The following chapters will discuss some of the basics that you need to know about the sugar detox diet. Most Americans take in too much sugar, much more than they need to function. And while these are causing a lot of bad health conditions, it can be impossible to get over the addiction since our bodies are predisposed to eat as much sugar as possible. The sugar detox is the solution that you need to help you get over this sugar addiction and get back to healthier and more nutritious eating.

Inside this guidebook, you will find all the information that you need to finally get started with the sugar detox. We will discuss some of the basics that come with this meal plan as well as the differences that are found in the three levels of this diet plan.

Once you have decided that the sugar detox is the solution that you are looking for, it is time to get started. And that is often the hardest step of them all. This guidebook will provide you with a complete menu plan plus all of the recipes that you need to get through the 21-day sugar detox and to see the results that you want. When you are done with these three short weeks, you will be set for all the healthy nutritional choices that you need.

When you are ready to get started on the sugar-free detox, make sure to read through this guidebook and gain all the tools that you need to be successful.

There are plenty of books on this subject on the market, thanks again for choosing this one! Every effort was made to ensure it is full of as much useful information as possible, please enjoy!

Chapter 1: What is the Sugar Detox and the Basics of the Levels?

The sugar detox is a basic diet plan that is meant to help reduce your addiction to sugar. Sugar is found all over our society today and it is easy to reach and grab almost any food at the grocery store, especially the frozen and pre-made varieties, and take in a ton of excess sugar. In fact, most Americans will take in four times the amount of sugar that they need to function.

Most Americans realize that sugar is bad for them. They know that they shouldn't take in too much sugar and all of the bad health effects that come with this excess sugar. But no matter how much they may try, those cravings for sugar can make it almost impossible to avoid reaching for a baked good or another source of sugar when you are stressed or when you need some comfort food.

The reason that it is so hard to go against the sugar cravings is that it is against our biology. During the Paleolithic period, those who were able to eat sugar were the ones more likely to survive. This is because sugar can help you to store more fat. When times are lean and it is hard to find food, the ability to store food can be so important to your survival and this helped our ancestors to stay alive.

The issue now is that while we still have that predisposition towards craving sugar, sugar is so easy to find everywhere we turn. Our ancestors were lucky to find a bit of fruit or honey on occasion and so it made sense that they would grab it up whenever they could. But with sugar so prevalent today, it is harder to avoid taking in too much sugar rather than too little.

And it is all this extra consumption of sugar that is making us so sick. Diabetes, heart disease, stroke, and obesity are all tied to our increased sugar intake. Many times, we may try to avoid taking in the sugar, but since sugars are found even in some healthy foods (think fruits and those "health" foods that sneak the sugar inside), it is hard to fight off those cravings.

This is where the 21-day sugar detox comes in. This detox is all about giving the body a break from that excess sugar so that it can concentrate on repairing itself and fighting off other toxins that may come into the body. On this detox, you will need to cut out all types of sugars, even most of the carbs that may be considered healthy. Outside of very low sugar fruits, vegetables, and gluten free grains, your carb intake will be low for this short period of time.

This may seem extreme, but it is meant to help you break off from your sugar addiction. If you are taking in sugars, even if they are the healthy sugars found in fruits and good carbs, it could still trigger you to reach for the other bad sugars that you should avoid. For the 21-days, you will cut out all carbs and sugars as much as possible so that your body can reset.

After the 21-days are over, you will be able to add back in some of the good carbs and the fruits. But since you have gone through these three weeks of the detox, you are set to make healthier and smarter food choices. You will be able to eat the sugars a few times a day and not go overboard. It is such a short period of time, but it can do wonders for fighting off your sugar cravings and helping you to get on a healthier diet plan.

Health issues with eating sugar

There are a lot of health issues that are associated with eating too much sugar. Remember that our bodies are programmed to take in more sugar because, in the past, this helped us to hold onto fat and get through the lean periods that could happen when food is scarce.

In modern times, sugar is not scarce and it is easy to get ahold of it any time that we want. We are able to find sugar in almost any of the foods that we want to eat, especially when we are looking at hidden sugars, and we end up taking in way more than we really need to. We end up overloading our bodies with all of these sugars, and it can make the body sick.

Those who take in too much sugar are going to face a variety of health conditions. Some of these include issues like:

- Obesity: obesity is pretty common when you are dealing with eating too much sugar. This is because when you consume sugar, you are likely eating a food choice that is high in calories. Then, a few hours later, you are going to feel hungry again. These high sugar foods are going to make you feel pretty hungry all of the time and you will take in way more calories than the body needs, making you gain weight quickly.

- Heart disease: one thing that surprises a lot of people is how much sugar is able to affect your heart health. Sugar has been linked to heart diseases like stroke, high blood pressure, and heart attacks.
- High blood pressure: high amounts of sugar, especially over time, will increase your blood pressure. The sugars that you consume will restrict the blood vessels, which will make it so the blood pushes against the arteries harder than before. It can be almost as bad on your body as eating too much sodium, and when you combine them together, which can happen with many of those junk foods you consume, you could be in for trouble.
- Diabetes: when we take in sugar, we end up raising our insulin levels. The insulin is in charge of breaking up the sugar and converting it into a substance that the cells are able to absorb. But when you start to take in too much sugar, the body becomes resistant to the insulin, or it can stop producing insulin in the first place. Both of these are side effects of diabetes. The sugar-free detox can help you to restore the body and stop the progression of diabetes.

The more sugar that you take in on a daily basis, the harder it will be to prevent some of these health conditions. Learning how to change your eating habits and cutting down the sugars that you consume will help you to get your health back on track.

Why are grains and fruit taken out of the diet?

One thing that you will notice when you first get started with the sugar-free detox is that pretty much all fruits and grains are going to be taken away from the diet. When it comes to the fruits, you are allowed to have one piece of a banana or an apple and then unlimited amounts of lemon and lime and still stay on the diet, no matter which option you choose. While fruits have the healthy sugars in them, the idea of the sugar-free detox is that you need to cut out as many sugars as you can. Fruits are high in sugars and you can get most of those nutrients from lower carb vegetables. The good news is that you can bring them back into your diet later on when the detox is all done.

In all of the levels of the sugar-free detox, you will have to reduce a number of grains that you take in. In the first level, you are allowed to have about half a cup of gluten free grains. This makes it a little bit easier to get started on the diet, but you will be surprised at how little half a cup can be. When you move into the later levels, you will even have to cut out more carbs going down to pretty much nothing. You will pretty much get your carbs from the healthy vegetables that are allowed on this diet plan.

Another thing that you will notice is that in the third level of this sugar detox, you will be required to cut out even the milk products. The first two allow these in moderate amounts because of the good fats and protein, as well as the calcium that is found in these products. But on the third level, you will cut out dairy products because they are high in lactose, the milk sugar. This is not necessarily unhealthy in small amounts, but the third level is about taking it to the next level and so you cut them out.

The reason that you take out these "healthy" foods is pretty simple. Getting over a sugar addiction can be hard. Taking in any amount of sugar, even if it is considered healthy sugars, can be detrimental to your results. These foods may be considered healthy for the body and may have some of the good nutrients that your body needs, but they also have nutrients that convert into sugar in the body. Getting rid of them for a short amount of time will make it easier to get rid of the sugar habit. Once you are done with the three weeks, you can slowly start to add these foods back in.

The levels of the sugar detox

When you start the 21-day detox, there are three levels that you are able to pick from. You will notice that they are very similar to each other, but there are a few key differences. Each of them will help you to see the results that you are looking for; it is more up to your personal preferences over what you would like to do. There are also some modifications that come with each of the levels. The 21-day detox will offer modifications for autoimmune issues, energy (if you work-out often you may want to go with this option), and the Pescetarian.

Level one is going to be the easiest level on this detox plan with the third level being the strictest. If you are not used to being on a diet of any kind or you have had trouble sticking with any in the past, level one is going to be the best option for you to choose. Keep in mind that the level you choose to go through during this 21-day detox is your choice.

Often, if this is your first time going through the 21-day detox, you will want to start with level one. And then if you decide to go through it again, you would pick level two and level three since these have a few more stringent guidelines that you will need to follow. All three levels can be effective for your results, they just present some different challenges from each other.

The modifications of the sugar detox

As mentioned a bit before, there are some modifications that are allowed on each part of the 21-day sugar detox. The most common modifications that you will find include those for autoimmune disorders, for added energy, and for pescetarian diets. The modifications are all created in order to make it easier to enhance your experience and make it more personal if you need to change some of your nutritional needs.

If you do decide that you need to go through one of these modifications, you need to follow them correctly. Otherwise, you are going to end up struggling more with the detox symptoms compared to doing it correctly. In addition, the Pescetarian modifications are not really appropriate for the food choices on level three because that level will cut out some of the foods that are needed for that modification to get the right nutrition. You have to remember that you have to pick the right level to go with your modifications as well.

Remember that the modifications and the levels together were created after many people finished the 21-day sugar detox. If you are choosing one of the harder levels just because you want fast results, and not because it is the best one for you, it may not yield the good results that you would like. You are also allowed to come back and do another round of this diet plan with some different levels or modifications, but make sure that you follow the yes and no lists as close as possible.

Simple tips to get started

While all of the levels are a little bit different, there are some things that you can keep in mind for all of the levels, no matter which one you choose. Some of the things that you should remember when you get started include:

- No added sweeteners: the only things that are sweet that you are allowed are those fruits that are on your Yes list for the level. If you see a food that has some kind of added sweetener in it, you are not allowed to consume it. The full-fat dairy that is allowed on the first two levels have sugar in them, and that is fine, as long as the total grams of carbs don't go above 1 gram.
- If the food item tastes sweet and you don't find it on your Limit or Yes list, you are not allowed to

consume it. If you are unsure about it and the food tastes sweet, don't eat it.

- Grain flours: you are not able to eat grain flours including refined-grains or whole-grains. The ones that are allowed would be those from coconut, seeds, and nuts and some starches are fine.
- If you are in doubt, always leave the food out.
- Stick with non-starchy vegetables: one of the main sources of carbs that you will enjoy on this diet plan are the non-starchy vegetables. Your Yes and No lists will include quite a few options; so, try and mix and match them a bit when you create your meals. These will provide you with all of the nutrients that the body needs as well as some healthy carbs that will give you energy on this diet plan. There are a few starchy ones you can include too, but try to keep these down to the minimum.
- Avoid most fruits: when you are on this diet plan, you should avoid most types of fruits because they are high in sugars that can trigger you to eat other bad carbs and sugars. You are allowed to have a little bit of fruit each day on this detox, but you need to read your Yes and No lists.
- Find a friend to do it with you: doing the diet on your own is sometimes hard. One way that you can make sure that you are sticking with the diet is to find a friend who will go on it with you. You can offer each other support along the way and be there to pick each other up when the need arises.
- Remember it is just three weeks: this detox plan is going to be really hard. Your body is going to carve all of those sugars that you gave up, and in

the first few days, you may feel a reaction for giving up the sugar, such as body aches, moodiness, and headaches. You will be giving up an addiction, and this can be hard to deal with. The important thing is to remember that this plan is only for three weeks. You can easily get through anything for three weeks and when the time is over, you are set to eat healthier options and change your eating habits.

Following the 21-day sugar detox is one of the best ways for you to fight off your sugar addiction and feel better in no time. It only takes three weeks to accomplish this goal and you will be able to enjoy good carbs without all the worry.

Chapter 2: A Look at Level One on the Sugar Detox

The first level that we are going to look at is level one of the sugar detox. This is considered one of the most lenient levels of the detox so if you are just getting started on this diet plan or you have never done a diet plan before, this is the best ones to choose. Remember that you are able to use the Yes and No Food Lists to create your own food plans or you can use the meal plan that is available in this guidebook.

The Yes List

In each of these levels, you will be able to find that there is a yes list, a limited list, and then a no list (which will include everything that is not on the other two lists). The following items are allowed on the yes list for the first level of this detox.

Whole grains (1/2 cup a day)

Tapioca
Sorghum
Rice (brown and wild)
Quinoa
Millet
Lentils
Garbanzo beans
Buckwheat

Beans
Arrowroot
Amaranth

If you are following a meal plan, consider where you need to place these carbs. Some people feel best if they are able to eat them earlier in the day to give them the energy to keep on moving, and others like to have it at night. You can always change around the meals to get the best results for you.

Full-Fat Dairy

This first level on the sugar detox will allow you to have some full-fat dairy products. You need to remember that you are not able to have options that have added sugars in them, but the natural lactose sugars found in these dairy products are just fine. Some of the full-fat dairy products that you can enjoy include:

Sour cream
Kefir or plain yogurt
Half and half
Heavy cream
Whole milk
Cottage cheese
Cream cheese
Cheese

Listen to your body to figure out how much dairy you are able to have. Some people find that they are sensitive to the milk products and will only include it in on occasion. You can add it into the diet each day or just occasionally.

Meat

Meat is allowed on this diet plan and in fact, it is encouraged while you are on this 21-day detox. You are able to eat all meats. This does include cured meats like prosciutto, pancetta, and bacon and deli meats are fine. All seafood is fine and so are eggs.

Vegetables

Non-starchy vegetables are just fine for you to enjoy. You can take in moderate amounts of these and in fact, during these three weeks, these vegetables will be one of your only sources of carbs on all the levels of this detox. Some of the healthy vegetables that are allowed include:

Kale
Jicama
Horseradish
Green beans
Ginger
Garlic
Eggplant
Cucumber
Collards
Chard
Celery and celery root
Carrots
Cabbage
Brussels sprouts
Broccoli
Asparagus

Artichokes
Zucchini
Yellow squash
Turnips
Tomato
Spinach
Spaghetti squash
Snap and snow peas
Rutabaga
Radishes
Radicchio
Peppers, any type
Parsnips
Onions
Mushrooms
All types of leafy greens
Leeks

Fruits

There are only two types of fruits that you are allowed to have in unlimited amounts in this diet plan. You are able to use these as a flavoring in your meals so they are great to use when you are not able to add sauces and other flavorings on your meals. The two fruits that you are able to eat include lime and lemon.

Nuts and seeds

Nuts and seeds are encouraged when you are on this diet plan and they can make for a great snack when you follow this detox. Remember that they need to be the regular variety; you are not able to add sugars or salt to them or you will kick them off the diet plan. Some of the nuts and seeds that you are allowed to eat include:

Pumpkin seeds
Pistachios
Pecans
Macadamia nuts
Hemp seeds
Flax seeds
Filberts or hazelnuts
Coconut (but you are not able to use coconut sugar)
Chia seeds
Cocoa
Brazil nuts
Almonds
Walnuts
Sesame seeds
Sunflower seeds

Fats and oils

One thing that you should not forget to add into the diet plan are the healthy fats and oils. These are needed to help you to stay healthy and will ensure that you are getting the good nutrition that you need to stay healthy. Some of the good fats and oils that you can enjoy include:

Sesame oil
Olives and olive oil
Flax oil
Coconut oil
Avocados and avocado oil

Butter or ghee
Animal fats

Condiments

You do need to be careful with the types of condiments that you choose to go with. You can have some, but you do have to watch out for those that have a lot of extra sugars inside of them. Some of the condiments that are fine for you to enjoy include:

Homemade Mayo
Hummus from cauliflower
Extracts including vanilla bean, almond, and vanilla
Coconut amino
Homemade broth
Mustard if it is gluten free
Brewer's yeast
Homemade salad dressings
Herbs and spices
Vinegar including rice, sherry, white, red wine, distilled, balsamic, and apple cider

Limited Foods

In addition to the foods that are in the list above, you will be able to have a few other types of foods, but you need to eat these in very limited quantities. These are going to include a few other fruits and some starchy vegetables, though you are not allowed to have as many of them as you would like. But if you need something a bit different on occasion on the detox, these can be just fine.

Starchy Vegetables (only 1 cup a day)

Green peas
Butternut squash
Beets
Acorn squash
Winter squash
Pumpkin

Fruit

You are only allowed to have one piece of these fruits each day. These have some more sugar in them than the lemon and the lime that you are able to enjoy so you do need to limit them a little bit. Some of the fruits that you are able to eat on occasion include:

Green and Granny Smith apples
Grapefruit
Bananas, ones that aren't quite ripe

Whole grains (1/2 cup a day)

Tapioca
Sorghum
Rice (brown and wild)
Quinoa
Millet
Lentils
Garbanzo beans
Buckwheat
Beans

Arrowroot
Amaranth

If you are following a meal plan, consider where you need to place these carbs. Some people feel best if they are able to eat them earlier in the day to give them the energy to keep on moving, and others like to have it at night. You can always change around the meals to get the best results for you.

Beverages

For the most part, you will want to stick with water, although some herbal teas and a bit of coffee are fine as well. Some of the other beverages that you are able to have, although you need to limit it to just 1 cup each day, include:

Kombucha, store bought or homemade
Coconut water and juice, as long as you don't add in sweeteners.

The No List

If you are searching through your Yes and Limited lists and you don't find a food that is on it, this means that you are not allowed to have any amount of these foods on this diet plan. It may be tempting, but you need to avoid these foods or you can ruin all your hard work with this diet plan.

This means that you will need to avoid all of the refined carbs, any of the vegetables that are on this list, most fruits, and so on. Just make sure to stick with the foods that are on the Yes and Limited list and you will do fine. Our meal plan later in this book will help you to get started with these tasty foods.

Remember that level one is considered the most lenient of the plans on the 21-day detox. This is a great one to get started on and will help you to get started while still providing some great results.

Chapter 3: A Look at Level Two on the Sugar Detox

In some cases, you may choose to get started on the second level of the 21-day sugar detox. This is a bit harder and more challenging option on the sugar detox, which makes it a good choice in a few ways. To start, if you have done the 21-day sugar detox in the past, starting another round on level two can be a great idea. This allows you to build upon what you have done in the past so that you continue to see results.

This level is going to be similar to what you found in the first level of the sugar detox, but there are a few changes that make this level a bit more challenging. There will also be a Yes and Limited list. Anything that does not end up on these two lists is not allowed when you are following the second level on this sugar detox.

If you are going to level two, you are able to use many of the same meals that are on our menu plan in this guidebook, but you can make some modifications as well. Some people like to go through the Yes and No food list and make up their own meal plans as well since this provides them with some more flexibility. The choice is all yours.

The biggest difference that you will notice on this part is that you need to cut out the whole grains that are allowed. In the first level, you were allowed to have half a cup of them each day, but on this version, you need to cut them out completely. The rest of the lists are going to stay the same as the first level.

Energy Modification

In level one and level two, you are allowed to make some modifications to help you get the results to personalize for your needs. The first one will be the energy modification or the one for those who will need more of the healthy carbs. You may need these modifications if you:

- Have a job that is physically demanding or work an active lifestyle.
- Participate in exercise or physical activity that is really high intensity. Yoga would not count by endurance athletics and Cross-Fit options would.
- You are nursing or pregnant.

The first thing that you can add into this plan are some starchy vegetables. You are able to add about 30 to 50 grams of these carbs to at least one of your meals each day, but make sure that you are adding them in shortly after exercising. This could be about half a cup of sweet potatoes that are allowed. Adding a piece of fruit works well. You will have to decide how much extra you are allowed to have based on how intensely.

There are some recommendations to help you learn how many extra carbs that you will need. These include:

- Moderately active: you can have about 75 extra grams of carbs each day.
- Highly active: can have up to 200 grams, but should probably stay under.
- Pregnant or nursing; get at least 100 grams each day.

Listen to your body at all times and figure out what is best for you. Most of the time you will be fine sticking with the basics of this diet and you don't need to make modifications. But those who are athletes or pregnant and nursing will need to get a bit more nutrition to help them out. In these cases, you still need to keep it pretty low and it is best to stick with some of the starchy vegetables, rather than adding more of the other carb options.

Pescetarian Modification

Another modification that you can do on this diet plan is to follow it while on a pescetarian diet. You will need to make some changes in the diet plan to ensure that you are getting the nutrition that your body needs. When you are following these types of modifications, you allowance of legumes and whole grains will increase. You can also add in some of the starchy vegetables to the meal plan even though they are placed on the No foods list.

On the pescetarian diet, you are able to have a maximum of two cups a day of the starchy vegetables. This would include some options like sweet potatoes, yams, potatoes, and more to help you get a bit more of the nutrition that you need. You can also add in some more high-quality dairy to your meals because these will help you to get more of the fat and protein that your body needs. When picking out the dairy products that you want to use, stick with the non-homogenized varieties and the grass-fed ones. If you aren't able to find the grass-fed options, you should go with organic.

Another thing that you should do is add in some extra fats. You can add in a bit during your meals and in your snacks. There are so many great ways that you are able to add in these extra fats including;

Add in a full avocado, rather than the half that is usually recommended.

Make use of your full-fat dairy so that you can get the right amount of protein and fat. If you find that you are not tolerating dairy all that well, such as dealing with gas, digestive distress, and bloating, you should cut these out and find other sources of fat.

And of course, you need to eat seafood as much as possible. This is going to provide you with a lot of the good protein that you need, especially since you won't be getting it from other options on this plan. You should have seafood for one meal each day, but it is best if you can fit it into two or more meals each day so that you get the amount of protein that the body needs.

Level two is going to be pretty similar to the first level, but you are going to be more limited on the grains that you are able to enjoy. If you are worried about this one being too restrictive, it is just fine for you to go ahead and stick with level one. All of these levels can be effective for you to see the results that you want, but you have to know your body and what will work the best for it.

Chapter 4: A Look at Level Three on the Sugar Detox

And finally, it is time to move on to level three. If you are just getting started on a sugar detox, especially if you have never gone on a diet plan in the past before, this is probably not the option that you will go with. It is the hardest of the three levels to work with and so it is best for those who really need to make some changes to their diet quickly, or those who have already done some rounds with the 21-day sugar detox in the beginning.

When you get started with the 21-day sugar detox, you will notice that there will be some similarities. You will find that some of the foods that are on the Yes and Limited lists will be the same, but the main differences are that there will be a few more items that are added to the No list compared to what is in the other two levels.

The point on this level is to help you really reduce the carbs and the sugars that you are consuming so that you can see the results that you want. If you are really addicted to sugar and are worried that even a bit will set you off to eating too much sugar, then this can be a good place to start. Or, those who have already done this diet a few times will like it because it helps them to get even further with their healthy eating.

With that being said, you should not choose the third level of this sugar detox because you are trying to challenge yourself too much, or just because you think it will give you better results, then this is not the right option for you. This one is tougher, but you won't necessarily see better results. It is just another level to help you out. If you are just starting and you are fine with a bit of the carb, level one is definitely the place where you need to get started.

As mentioned, level three is going to be the most difficult of the three levels to complete with level one being the easiest. But one of the first questions that you may have is how is this third level so different from the first and the second level?

In level one, you were allowed to have some grains. They were going to be really limited, just down to half a cup each day and that is all, but you were still allowed to have them. In both level one and level two, you are allowed to have some dairy, as long as you stick with the whole fat dairy products and you pick out options that are not going to have added sugars in them.

But when you are on level three of the sugar detox, you will need to exclude both the grains and all of the dairy products. This version of the sugar-free detox is sometimes known as the Paleo version. There are some differences between the Paleo diet and the third level of this detox though. In the third level, you are also supposed to kick out all of the sweet tasting foods and the excess natural sugars, all of those except the ones found in your limited fruits and some vegetables, from your diet while some of these are allowed on the Paleo diet.

This version is going to seem a bit extreme to some people, but the point is to help you reduce all of the sweet foods that you may rely on in the past and it is in charge of changing some of your habits. For some people, having even a bit of natural sweetener or the sugars that come in natural grains and dairy will set them off and make it so that they want to have more of these foods or other bad options. Level three takes away some of that temptation by eliminating even these foods so that you get as little sugar in the diet as possible for the three weeks.

It is going to be hard, but for the really bad sugar addictions, it is the one that you should go with. Or if you have tried the diet in the past, it is another method to try to see results. You only have to stick with it for three weeks, and then you can add back in some of the dairy products, healthy grains, and so on to see results.

Outside of the whole grains and the dairy products that were mentioned before, you will be able to follow the Yes, Limited, and No lists that were available for the other two options. Make sure to get in plenty of healthy protein to help you stay healthy and don't forget those great fats that will provide you with good nutrition. You are still able to eat the non-starchy vegetables that you would like, but keep the fruits down to just the few that are listed.

Following one of the three levels for the sugar detox will help you to see the results that you would like. Each of them can be critical to helping you get rid of your sugar addiction and start eating healthier meals. You can choose the one that is right for your needs. All of them can be successful, so, don't stress if you need to go with the first level to give it a try, you are still going to see some results.

Chapter 5: Your 21-Day Meal Plan to Kickstart Your Results

While the ideas behind the sugar-free detox are pretty simple, there are some steps that need to happen before you can really start to see results with it. One of the hardest things to work on is finding the foods that you can eat on this diet and ensure that you can meal plan without spending hours in the process.

The good news is that this diet plan is only 21 days. That is all it takes to help you get started on healthier eating habits that include cutting out the sugar. But once you are done with these simple three weeks, you will be set to eat a healthier and more nutritious lifestyle for many years to come.

This chapter is going to be your best friend when you start the sugar detox. This chapter will provide you with a 21-day meal plan, long enough to get you through the whole detox, so you can set yourself up for success right from the beginning!

Day 1

Breakfast: Morning Muffins
Lunch: Tuna Salad
Dinner: Beef Muffins
Snack

Day 2:

Breakfast: Pancakes
Lunch: Tomato Salad
Dinner: Mushroom Pizza
Snack: Apple Turnovers

Day 3

Breakfast: Crème Cheese Crepes
Lunch: Tomato Soup
Dinner: Lamb Burgers
Snack: Healthy Crackers

Day 4

Breakfast: Breakfast Momo
Lunch: Parmesan Marinara
Dinner: Fish Fingers
Snack: Kale Chips

Day 5

Breakfast: Quick French Toast
Lunch: Chicken Buffalo Salad
Dinner: Kung Pao Chicken
Snack: Avocado Tortillas

Day 6

Breakfast: Egg Whites
Lunch: Mushroom Soup
Dinner: Prawn Courgetti
Snack: Cream Cheese Snacks

Day 7

Breakfast: Vanilla Yogurt
Lunch: Beef and Cabbage
Dinner: Green Bean Casserole
Snack: Whole Food Bars

Day 8

Breakfast: Almond Squares
Lunch: Egg Frittata
Dinner: Eggplant Lasagna
Snack: Goji Bars

Day 9

Breakfast: Coconut Pudding
Lunch: Parmesan Marinara
Dinner: Chicken Stir-Fry
Snack: Cashew Butter Balls

Day 10

Breakfast: Cinnamon Cereal
Lunch: Chicken Cashew Salad
Dinner: Peach Chicken
Snack: Apple Turnovers

Day 11

Breakfast: Chia Breakfast
Lunch: Grilled Salmon
Dinner: Shrimp and Spinach
Snack: Healthy Crackers

Day 12

Breakfast: Cream Cheese Crepes
Lunch: Mango Chicken
Dinner: Spicy Chicken
Snack: Kale Chips

Day 13

Breakfast: Pancakes
Lunch: Moroccan Chicken
Dinner: Cheesy Zucchini Bake
Snack: Pecan Delight

Day 14

Breakfast: Almond Pudding
Lunch: Lamb Ragu
Dinner: Mongolian Beef
Snack: Avocado Tortillas

Day 15

Breakfast: Morning Muffins
Lunch: Tuna Salad
Dinner: Beef Muffins
Snack: Cream Cheese Snacks

Day 16

Breakfast: Breakfast Momo
Lunch: Mushroom Soup
Dinner: Lamb Burgers
Snack: Whole Food Bars

Day 17

Breakfast: Egg Whites
Lunch: Chicken Buffalo Salad
Dinner: Mushroom Pizza
Snack: Goji Bars

Day 18

Breakfast: Coconut Pudding
Lunch: Grilled Salmon
Dinner: Fish Fingers
Snack: Cashew Butter Balls

Day 19

Breakfast: Quick French Toast
Lunch: Mango Chicken
Dinner: Eggplant Lasagna
Snack: Whole Food Bars

Day 20

Breakfast: Pancakes
Lunch: Egg Frittata
Dinner: Kung Pao Chicken
Snack: Goji Bars

Day 21

Breakfast: Almond Squares
Lunch: Lamb Ragu
Dinner: Peach Chicken
Snack: Cashew Butter Balls

Chapter 6: Starting Your Day with a Great Breakfast Recipes

Breakfast is one of the most important meals of the day and starting your day with something that is good and healthy, without being loaded with sugars, can help you to feel full, satisfied, and energetic for the day. Here are some of the great recipes that you need to follow with the meal plan or mix and match them to meet your needs.

Almond Pudding

Ingredients:

- Peach (half)
- Almond flour (4 Tbsp.)
- Cinnamon (1 pinch)
- Almonds (6)
- Almond milk (1 c.)

How it's made:

- Pour the almond milk and flour into your pressure cooker. Stir in the cinnamon
- Add the lid on top and cook for a few minutes.
- Allow the mixture to cool. Chop up the peaches and add them to the top.
- Garnish with the almonds and serve.

Chia Breakfast

Ingredients:

- Hot water (0.6 c.)
- Flax meal (0.75 c.)
- Coconut milk (2 Tbsp.)
- Chia seeds (0.75 c.)
- Coconut (0.75 c)
- Cinnamon (1 tsp.)

How it's made:

- Mix the chia seeds, coconut sugar, coconut, cinnamon, and flax meal together.
- Divide up into some serving bowls when mixed.
- Add in the amount of coconut milk you need and mix.
- Eat four minutes later.

Cinnamon Cereal

Ingredients:

- Cinnamon (1 Tbsp.)
- Chia seeds (.25 c.)
- Coconut (1 c.)
- Salt (.5 tsp.)
- Stevia (.25 c.)
- Egg (1)
- Sunflower seeds (.5 c.)

How it's made:

- Ensure that the oven heats up to 325 degrees.
- Low out some parchment paper on a baking sheet.
- Place the cinnamon, sunflower seeds, chia seeds, salt, and coconut in your blender. Turn it on for 30 seconds.
- Whisk the egg and the coconut mixture in a bowl and mix the stevia.
- Add this to the baking sheet and put into the oven.
- Take out 20 minutes later and serve in a bowl with milk.

Coconut Pudding

Ingredients:

- Coconut milk (2 c.)
- Nuts as topping
- Shredded coconut (.5 c.)
- Chia seeds (.25 c.)

How it's made:

- Add some coconut milk into a bowl and soak your chia seed to it.
- After ten minutes, add in the coconut. Cover with plastic wrap and place in the fridge.
- Add a few nuts on top before serving.

Almond Squares

Ingredients:

- Melted dark chocolate (4.5 oz.)
- Coconut oil (2 Tbsp.)
- Stevia (0.75 c.)
- Melted almond butter (1 c.)
- Almond flour (0.75 c.)
- Coconut (0.75 c)

How it's made:

- Place the almond flour, coconut, and stevia in a bowl.
- In a separate bowl, mix the coconut oil and melted butter. Pour this into the flour mixture.
- Once this is well mixed, spread it out onto a prepared tray.
- Melt the chocolate and pour it over the rest of the mixture.
- Place everything into the freezer for a minimum of 4 hours.

Vanilla Yogurt

Ingredients:

- Vanilla (1 tsp.)
- Warm water (.5 c.)
- Almond milk (.75 c)
- Chia seeds (2 Tbsp.)
- Stevia (2 Tbsp.)
- Almonds (1 c.)

How it's made:

- Lay out the almonds in a bowl and pour some almonds on top of them. Leave this alone for the next 4 hours. Drain out the water through a strainer.
- During this time, pour some water into another bowl and soak your chia seeds another 20 minutes.
- After everything is soaked, take out the blender and pulse the almond milk, vanilla, stevia, and almonds.
- Blend this well and add in the chia to mix more.
- Add some plastic wrap or a lid to the bowl you are using and place in the fridge for six hours.

Egg Whites

Ingredients:

- Chopped onion (.5 c.)
- Pepper
- Salt
- Bell pepper (.25 c.)
- Egg whites (1 c.)
- Chopped spinach (.25 c)

How it's made:

- Ensure that the oven heats up to 375 degrees. Use some cooking spray to prepare your muffin tin.
- Add a spoon of the egg whites into each part of the muffin tins.
- When the eggs are ready, add the spinach, bell pepper, and onions, keeping everything even.
- Season with the pepper and salt and then place into the oven.
- Twenty minutes later, take the eggs out and serve.

Quick French Toast

Ingredients:

- Egg whites (.3 c.)
- Vanilla (.5 tsp.)
- Bread, low carb (4 pieces)
- Stevia (.5 Tbsp.)
- Almond milk (1 Tbsp.)
- Cinnamon
- Egg (1)

How it's made:

- Use a whisk to beat the egg whites. Add in the rest of the eggs and keep on beating.
- When that is done, add in the cinnamon, Stevia, hazelnut, almond milk, and vanilla.
- Once the mixture is done, take the bread and dip on both sides into this mixture.
- Fry the bread in a skillet.
- Repeat these steps with the rest of your bread and then serve.

Breakfast Momo

Ingredients:

- Tomato puree (1 tsp.)
- Diced onion (4)
- Salt
- Diced green chilies (2)
- Shrimp (1 c.)
- Water (.5 c)
- Olive oil (1 Tbsp.)
- Almond flour (1 c.)

How it's made;

- Bring out the shrimp and slice into small pieces. Add into a bowl with the tomato puree.
- Once the shrimp are covered, add the salt, chilies, and onion. Leave this alone for about 10 minutes.
- In your second bowl, combine your water and flour to make a dough. Roll it out and make lots of little circles.
- Remove these circles and add your shrimp mixture to each round. Fold the rounds to the middle and seal it up.
- Add a bit of water to the pressure cooker and add in a trivet.
- Add these rounds to a steaming basket and place into the pressure cooker.
- Ten minutes later, serve these hot.

Cream Cheese Crepes

Ingredients:

- Butter (1 tsp.)
- Soft cream cheese (3 oz.)
- Stevia (1 Tbsp.)
- Beaten egg (2)
- Cinnamon (1 tsp.)

How it's made:

- Beat the cream cheese and eggs together so they become smooth. Add in the cinnamon and the syrup.
- Once everything has time to mix, leave the mixture alone for a bit.
- Ten minutes later, melt some butter in a pan.
- Work in batches and fry the crepes before serving.

Pancakes

Ingredients:

- Egg whites (1)
- Sugar-free Jell-O (1 packet)
- Almond flour (1 c.)
- Egg (1)

How it's made:

- Throw your egg white and egg together and beat them together.
- When those are done, add in the almond flour and your Jell-O and mix well.
- In your skillet, add in some butter and add a bit of the batter.
- Fry for a bit until both sides are browned. Continue with the rest of the batter and serve.

Morning Muffins

Ingredients:

- Olive oil (2 Tbsp.)
- Eggs (2)
- Salt
- Almond meal flour (.5 c.)
- Baking powder (.25 tsp.)
- Stevia (3 tsp.)
- Cinnamon (.5 tsp.)
- Coconut flour (1 c.)

How it's made:

- Ensure that the oven heats up to 350 degrees.
- The coconut flour, salt, almond meal, and baking powder need to mix together in a bowl.
- When those are done, add in the egg, oil, and stevia.
- Make sure this turns into a batter and pour into your muffin pan.
- Take the muffin tin and place into the oven.
- Ten minutes later, take out of the oven and enjoy.

Chapter 7: Beat the Afternoon Drag with These Healthy Lunch Recipes

Tuna Salad

Ingredients:

- Pepper
- Salt
- Mint (1 bunch)
- Oil (1 Tbsp.
- Crumbled feta (20 g.)
- Lemon juice (1 lemon)
- Tuna (1 c.)

How it's made:

- Slice up the tuna and add it to the skillet with some oil. Grill for five minutes.
- Throw the feta cheese, mint, pepper, and salt into a bowl before topping with the tuna.
- Drizzle with the lemon juice and mix around before serving.

Tomato Salad

Ingredients:

- Olive oil (1 Tbsp.)
- Sliced shallot (1)
- Pepper
- Balsamic vinegar
- Torn basil leaves (6)
- Sliced tomato (5 pieces)

How it's made:

- Your basil, shallot, and tomato should be thrown into a bowl. Mix in with the seasoning.
- Drizzle in the oils and use it to coat everything else before serving.

Chicken Buffalo Salad

Ingredients:

- Diced celery stalk (8)
- Buffalo wing sauce (1.5 Tbsp.)
- Mayo (3 Tbsp.)
- Boiled eggs (6)
- Blue cheese (.25 c.)
- Chicken thighs (6 oz.)

How it's made:

- Dice up the eggs and place inside of a bowl.
- Use your mayo to make into a paste before adding the blue cheese, wing sauce, and celery.
- Before serving, add in your chicken and toss a bit.

Tomato Soup

Ingredients:

- Chopped celery (1.5 c)
- Bay leaf (1)
- Sugar (1 Tbsp.)
- Dried oregano (1 tsp.)
- Water (2 c.)
- Olive oil (1 Tbsp.)
- Vegetable broth (2 c.)
- Onion (1 c.)
- Minced garlic cloves (2)
- Tomatoes (2 c.)
- Green bell pepper (1 c.)
- Parsley (.3 c.)
- Salt
- Diced green beans (1 c.)
- Pepper (.25 tsp.)

How it's made:

- Add some oil and the onion to a pot and fry it up. Add in the spices, herbs, and vegetables as well.
- When those are heated, pour in the broth and water.
- This meal needs to cook for an hour.
- Right before serving, add in some sugar and finish cooking.

Mushroom Soup

Ingredients:

- Salt
- Chopped onion (.6 c.)
- Truffle oil (1 tsp.)
- Thyme (.25 tsp.)
- Pepper
- Chopped mushrooms (2 c.)
- Milk (.5 c.)
- Flour (.25 c)
- Chicken broth (2 c.)
- Butter (1 Tbsp.)
- Bay leaf (1)

How it's made

- Inside of your pot fry up the onion and the butter.
- When the onion is fried, add in the mushrooms and go for another 3 minutes.
- Now you should toss in the flour, pepper, salt, milk, thyme, and bay leaf.
- This meal needs to cook for an hour and then serve hot.

Beef and Cabbage

Ingredients:

- Diced leafy greens (4 Tbsp.)
- Cashew butter (3 Tbsp.)
- Shredded green cabbage (1.5 c.)
- Salt (1 tsp.)
- Pepper (.25 tsp.)
- Italian seasoning (2 Tbsp.)
- Vinegar (1 Tbsp.)
- Shredded cheese (2 Tbsp.)
- Onion powder (1 tsp.)
- Beef (2 c.)

How it's made:

- Ensure that the air fryer heats up to 300 degrees.
- Using your wok, melt up the butter and then add in the beef to cook until done.
- Add the cabbage and cook a bit longer before adding in the remainder of the ingredients.
- When the cheese is melted, serve warm.

Parmesan Marinara

Ingredients:

- Mozzarella cheese (.5 c)
- Salt (.5 tsp.)
- Olive oil (2 Tbsp.)
- Minced garlic cloves (6)
- Marinara sauce (1 c.)
- Broccoli (1 head)

How it's made:

- Take the broccoli and cut it into smaller bits.
- Add together the olive oil, garlic, salt, and marinara. Add in your small bits of broccoli and toss around.
- Add the juice and the broccoli bits into a wok and cook a bit. When five minutes are up, add in the mozzarella to the top.
- Serve warm.

Egg Frittata

Ingredients:

- Olive oil (2 Tbsp.)
- Eggs (4)
- Paprika (1 tsp.)
- Turmeric (1 tsp.)
- Cumin (1 tsp.)
- Sliced capsicum, yellow (1)
- Sliced capsicum, red (1)
- Salt (1 tsp.)
- Sliced capsicum, green (1)

Directions:

- The eggs need to be added to a bowl and beaten so they become fluffy.
- Once the eggs are done, mix in the cumin, salt, paprika, and turmeric.
- Slowly add in your capsicum, the red, yellow, and green.
- Your wok needs to be heated up with some oil before pouring in the egg mixture.
- After five minutes of cooking, serve this warm.

Grilled Salmon

Ingredients:

- Pepper
- Salt
- Vinegar (1 Tbsp.)
- Olive oil (2 Tbsp.)
- Diced shallot (1)
- Basil leaves (.5 c)
- Toasted almonds (.25 c.
- Quartered cherry tomatoes (200 g)
- Salmon fillets (2)

How it's made:

- Use the pepper and salt to season the salmon.
- Heat up your oil and then fry your prepared salmon. After three minutes on both sides, take the fish out of the pan and let it cool down.
- Cube the salmon. While that cools down, combine the almonds, shallots, basil, and tomatoes.
- Add in the cubes of salmon and toss around.
- You will need another bowl to combine the rest of the ingredients. Pour into the original mixture and toss around.

Chicken Cashew Salad

Ingredients:

- Lemon zest (.5 tsp.)
- Lemon juice (1 Tbsp.)
- Olive oil (1 Tbsp.)
- Chopped cashews (2 Tbsp.)
- Pepper
- Soy sauce (1 Tbsp.)
- Yogurt (.5 c.)
- Salt (.25 tsp.)
- Chicken breasts (2)

How it's made:

- The chicken needs to marinate in the pepper, lemon juice, and soy sauce before beginning.
- After 30 minutes, place the chicken on the grill and cook until it is done. Slice up the chicken.
- Add the rest of the ingredients into a bowl and toss around before serving.

Mango Chicken

Ingredients:

- Pepper
- Salt
- Curry paste (1 Tbsp.)
- Toasted almond flakes (2 Tbsp.)
- Mango chutney (2 Tbsp.)
- Yogurt (4 Tbsp.)
- Sliced apricots (1 c.)
- Diced red pepper (1)
- Chopped spring onions (6)
- Sliced celery sticks (4)
- Chicken breast (2)

How it's made:

- For this recipe, slice the chicken into cubes and leave in a bowl.
- In the same bowl, add in the yogurt, curry paste, mango chutney, apricots, red pepper, onion, and celery.
- Season it a bit and then add in the almonds to serve.

Moroccan Chicken

Ingredients:

- Minced garlic clove (1)
- Diced red onion (1)
- Diced red bell pepper (2)
- Pepper
- Salt
- Red pepper flakes (.25 tsp)
- Cherry tomatoes (1 c.)
- Olive oil (1 Tbsp.)
- Chicken breasts (1 lb.)
- *Moroccan spice mix*
- Paprika (2 tsp.)
- Honey (2 tsp.)
- Olive oil (2 Tbsp.)
- Cumin (1 tsp.)
- Minced garlic clove (1)
- Cayenne pepper (1 pinch)
- Salt
- Ginger (.25 tsp.)
- Coriander (.5 tsp.)
- Cinnamon (.25 tsp.)
- Turmeric (.25 tsp.)

How it's made:

- Add all of the ingredients for the spice mix to a blender and puree. Move to a bowl and place the chicken inside.
- 30 minutes later, take the chicken out of the bowl and add to a pressure cooker.
- Add in the rest of the ingredients before cooking.
- After 30 minutes, serve the dish.

Lamb Ragu

Ingredients:

- Chopped thyme (.5 tsp.)
- Diced yellow onion (.5)
- Minced garlic clove (1)
- Diced celery rib (.5)
- Ground lamb (1 lb.)
- Chicken broth (.5 c.)
- Diced tomatoes (2 c.)
- Tomato paste (.5 Tbsp.)
- Cumin (1 tsp.)
- Red pepper flakes (.25 tsp.)
- Chopped rosemary (.5 tsp.)
- Sliced celery root (1)
- Olive oil (.5 tsp.)
- Pepper
- Salt
- Diced carrot (.5)

How it's made:

- Set up the pressure cooker and add in the celery, red pepper flakes, carrots, onion, cumin, pepper, rosemary, salt, garlic, thyme, and lamb.
- Cover and turn the heat on.
- After 20 minutes, add the chicken broth and tomato paste and cook a bit longer.
- Heat up the oil and the celeriac in a skillet for a few minutes and set to the side.
- After the lamb has cooked for 30 minutes, serve warm.

Chapter 8: Bring the Family Together for Dinner Recipes

Beef Muffins

Ingredients:

- Salt (.25 tsp.)
- Beef (3 c.)
- Almond milk (2 Tbsp.)
- Pepper (.25 tsp.)
- Diced onion (1 c.)
- Red bell pepper, diced (1 c.)
- Eggs (8)

How it's made:

- Ensure that the oven heats up to 350 degrees and use some liners to prepare the muffin tin.
- The eggs need to be beaten until they become fluffy.
- When the eggs are done, add the bell pepper, onion, almond milk, and beef, seasoning it all as well.
- Pour this beef and egg mixture into the muffin cups and put inside your hot oven.
- Ten minutes later, take it out and serve.

Mushroom Pizza

Ingredients:

- Olive oil (1 Tbsp.)
- Pepper
- Sat
- Sliced mushrooms (6)
- Salmon (.5 c)
- Cheese (.5 c)
- Diced avocado (1 c.)
- Tortilla (1)

How it's made:

- Ensure that the oven heats up to 350 degrees. Take out a tray and add in some parchment paper and your tortilla.
- Arrange out your avocado, mushroom, and salmon on top and sprinkle with the cheese.
- Drizzle with the olive oil and place in the oven.
- Take the pan out after five minutes and serve the pizza warm.

Lamb Burgers

Ingredients:

- Pepper
- Salt
- Feta cheese (.3 c)
- Soy sauce (1 Tbsp.)
- Avocado oil (.25 c.)
- Onion (.3 c.)
- Ground lamb (1 lb.)

How it's made:

- Your pepper, salt, cheese, soy sauce, onion, and lamb need to be mixed together.
- When these are mixed, use your hands to turn them into patties.
- Heat up the oil in a skillet and add the patties.
- Fry up the patties until they are done and serve.

Fish Fingers

Ingredients:

- Olive oil
- Cheddar cheese (1 Tbs.)
- Whole meal bread (.24 c)
- Smoked paprika (2 tsp.)
- Eggs (2)
- Salmon (4 lbs.)

How it's made:

- Take the fish and makeup ten pieces.
- Whisk your egg with the seasonings and set aside.
- Now we can work on the bread crumb. Add some oil to the cheese and the bread and place in a blender. Place out on a tray when well mixed.
- Dip the ten fish pieces first into the egg mixture and then coat with the bread mixture.
- Ensure that the oven reaches 400 degrees.
- Place the fish into the oven and after 20 minutes, take them out and serve.

Kung Pao Chicken

Ingredients:

- Snow peas (1 c.)
- Red bell pepper (1 c.)
- Red pepper (1 tsp.)
- Minced ginger (.5 tsp.)
- Brown sugar (1 tsp.)
- Cornstarch (2 tsp.)
- Soy sauce (3 Tbsp.)
- Water (.75 c.)
- Chicken thighs (1 lb.)
- Minced garlic clove (2)
- Chopped onion (1 c.)
- Sesame oil (2 Tbsp.)
- Peanuts (2 Tbsp.)

How it's made:

- Bring out your pan and heat up the garlic, onion, and oil to fry for about three minutes.
- Cook the chicken another 5 minutes and then move to a plate.
- Combine everything except the nuts, peas, and pepper and then add some water, about three cups.
- Stir around to dissolve the sugar before adding the peas and the pepper and finish cooking.
- Pour these ingredients into a bowl and top with the chicken and the nuts before serving.

Prawn Courgetti

Ingredients:

- Pine nuts (20 g.)
- Olive oil
- Diced red chili (.5)
- Minced garlic clove (1)
- Courgettes (3)
- Cherry tomatoes (.5 c.)
- Lemon zest (1)
- Lemon juice (1)
- King prawns (.5 c.)

How it's made:

- Ensure that the oven heats up to 400 degrees.
- Take out your baking tray and layer on the tomatoes. Place into the oven and then seven minutes later take it out.
- In a bowl add half the lemon juice and zest with the prawns and the pepper and salt. Toss and leave alone.
- Slice up your courgette into strips.
- When the prawns are ready, heat up some oil and fry them with the chili and the garlic.
- Add in the rest of the ingredients and then serve warm.

Green Bean Casserole

Ingredients:

- Flour (2 Tbsp.)
- Cooking spray
- Pepper
- Salt
- Skim milk (.75 c.)
- Cream of mushroom soup (1 c.)
- Onion (1)
- Mushrooms (1 pint)
- Green beans (2 c.)

Ho it's made:

- Ensure that the oven heats up to 400 degrees.
- Take your onion and let it become coated with the pepper, salt, and flour.
- Add the onions to a pan and place into the oven. In 15 minutes, take them out.
- Heat up some oil and fry up the cooked onions with the mushrooms a bit.
- Add in the mushroom soup, milk, and green beans. Cook another ten minutes.
- Pour all of this into a baking dish and place into the oven.
- Take out of the oven in thirty minutes and enjoy.

Eggplant Lasagna

Ingredients:

- Lasagna noodles (8 oz.)
- Cooking spray
- Ricotta cheese (1 c.)
- Basil (1 c.)
- Tomatoes (1 can)
- Red pepper (.25 tsp.)
- Oregano (.5 tsp.)
- Pepper (.75 tsp.)
- Chopped garlic cloves (3)
- Onion (.75 c.)
- Olive oil (2 tsp.)
- Salt (.75 tsp.)
- Eggplant (1)
- Mozzarella cheese (1 c.)
- Sliced zucchini (2)

How it's made:

- Ensure that the oven heats up to 350 degrees. Take out a dish and lay out the eggplant in one layer. Let it stand with some salt over it.
- Heat up the oil so that you can fry your garlic and onion. Add the salt, red pepper, oregano, and tomatoes.
- After ten minutes, move over to a bowl with the basil and ricotta.
- Add all of this to the dish from earlier.
- Add a layer of noodles, then some zucchini and some cheese and repeat.
- Place in the oven. After 35 minutes, take out of the oven and enjoy.

Chicken Stir-Fry

Ingredients:

- Diced onions (4)
- Salt
- Herbs
- Turmeric (2 Tbsp.)
- Soy sauce (2 Tbsp.)
- Olive oil (4 Tbsp.)
- Green chilies (3)
- Zucchini, diced (1 c.)
- Diced chicken breasts (4)

How it's made:

- Heat up the skillet with some oil. The chicken needs to be seared inside.
- After 5 minutes, add the soy sauce, zucchini, turmeric, and onion. Season a bit.
- Let it go for ten minutes on a lower heat before serving.

Peach Chicken

Ingredients:

- Salt (1 tsp.)
- Rose water (1 tsp.)
- Pepper
- Butter (.25 c.)
- Toasted almonds (.5 c.)
- Honey (.25 c.)
- Chicken (4 lb.)
- Peaches (1 lb.)

How it's made:

- Peel your peaches and slice up. Slice up the chicken as well.
- Ensure that the oven will heat up to 425 degrees.
- In a bowl, combine the pepper, rose water, salt, honey, and butter. Place in the microwave for 30 minutes.
- Add the chicken and coat well. Place on your baking tray and into the oven.
- After 15 minutes, take the chicken out. Add the peach slices and put back inside the oven.
- After 2 more minutes, take the chicken out.
- Top with the almonds.

Shrimp and Spinach

Ingredients:

- Crushed garlic cloves (2)
- Diced onion (1)
- Green chilies
- Pepper
- Olive oil (1 Tbsp.)
- Salt
- Soy sauce (1 Tbsp.)
- Shrimp (.3 c.)
- Spinach (1 c.)

How it's made:

- Start by preparing the shrimp. Add in some oil to the skillet and fry your garlic and onion for a bit.
- Add in the shrimp and then after five minutes add the soy sauce and the green chilies.
- Finally, add in the spinach and let it wilt before serving warm.

Spicy Chicken

Ingredients:

- Parsley (2 tsp.)
- Minced garlic clove (1)
- Chicken broth (.25 c.)
- Spicy green pepper sauce (3 Tbsp.)
- Pepper
- Salt
- Cubed chicken (1 breast)
- Minced shallot (1)

How it's made:

- Slice the chicken and add into a bowl with the pepper sauce to marinate. Put inside the fridge.
- After 30 minutes, take out. Add the garlic to a pan and fry a bit. Add in the shallots and the chicken and cook.
- After five minutes, add the broth and let it all cook for another ten minutes.
- Top with parsley and enjoy.

Cheesy Zucchini Bake

Ingredients:

- Parmesan cheese (2 Tbsp.)
- Salt (.5 tsp.)
- Cheddar cheese (8 oz.)
- Olive oil (2 Tbsp.)
- Quinoa (1 c.)
- Sliced zucchini (4 c.)

How it's made?

- Ensure that the oven is able to heat up to 400 degrees.
- Combine together the parmesan, cheddar cheese, salt, oil, zucchini, and quinoa (c0ok the quinoa if not done yet.)
- Pour this into your baking dish and then place in the oven.
- After 25 minutes, take the dish out and serve.

Mongolian Beef

Ingredients:

- Pepper
- Salt
- Soy sauce (.5 c.)
- Olive oil (1 Tbsp.)
- Cornstarch (2 Tbsp.)
- Chopped ginger (.5 tsp.)
- Minced garlic cloves (3)
- Diced onions (3)
- Water (.5 c)
- Steak (2 lbs.)

How it's made:

- Take the steak and add in some pepper and salt to it. In your skillet, cook the oil and steak for five minutes both sides.
- After this time, add the soy sauce, onion, garlic, and ginger.
- After three minutes, add in the cornstarch and mix together.
- Cook another ten minutes before serving.

Chapter 9: Snacks to Keep You on Track Recipes

Apple Turnovers

Ingredients:

- Cinnamon (1 tsp.)
- Vanilla (1 tsp.)
- Honey (1 c.)
- Milk (1 Tbsp.)
- Water (4 c.)
- Honey (4 Tbsp.)
- Lemon juice (2 Tbsp.)
- Butter (2 Tbsp.)
- Pastry sheets (1)
- Diced and peeled apples (4)

How it's made:

- Ensure that the oven is heated to 400 degrees.
- Add the lemon juice and water to a bowl with the apples to soak.
- After ten minutes, take the apples out and drain.
- Bring out a pot and add in the cinnamon, honey, milk, butter, and vanilla. Let this heat up.
- After five minutes add to a bowl and then use this to coat the apples.
- Lay out the pastry sheets and cut into squares.
- Add some of the apple mixture to the squares and then seal them up.
- Place onto the baking tray and then into the oven. After 10 minutes, take out of the oven and serve.

Healthy Crackers

Ingredients:

- Olive oil (1 Tbsp.)
- Water (1 Tbsp.)
- Egg (1)
- Flax seed (.5 c.)
- Tapioca flour (.5 c)
- Coconut oil (1 tsp.)

How it's made:

- Ensure that the oven heats up to 350 degrees and place some parchment paper on your baking sheet.
- Mix together the egg, flaxseed, and tapioca flour until they are well combined, adding some water as needed.
- Using your hands, add in the oil and knead the dough a bit. Roll it out and cut into squares with your knife.
- Place these squares on a baking sheet and then into the oven.
- After ten minutes, take the crackers out. Serve when cooled down a bit.

Kale Chips

Ingredients:

- Garlic salt (1 pinch)
- Pepper
- Coconut oil (1 Tbsp.)
- Kale leaves (1 bunch)

How it's made:

- Ensure that the oven heats up to 450 degrees.
- Tear up the kale leaves so they are in pieces and coat with some of the oil.
- Arrange this out on a tray and sprinkle with the pepper and garlic salt.
- Place into the warm oven. After 12 minutes, take the chips out and enjoy.

Pecan Delight

Ingredients:

- Salt (1 tsp.)
- Pecans (1 lb.)
- Water (1 Tbsp.)
- Cinnamon (1 tsp.)
- Honey (2 Tbsp.)
- Egg white (1)

How it's made:

- Ensure that the oven heats up to 250 degrees. During this time, whisk the egg white to make it frothy.
- Add in the rest of the ingredients before pouring on the baking tray.
- Place into the oven to warm up. After 12 minutes, take out from the oven and serve.

Avocado Tortillas

Ingredients:

- Honey (1 Tbsp.)
- Peanut butter (2 Tbsp.)
- Avocado (1)
- Tortilla, low carb (1)
- Raisins (2 Tbsp.)

How it's made

- Peel up the avocado and get rid of the pit before slicing up.
- Spread the peanut butter on the tortilla before topping with the raisins and avocado.
- Roll up your tortilla and add on more raisins. Cut in half and enjoy.

Cream Cheese Snacks

Ingredients:

- Jalapeno peppers (20)
- Mayo (.25 c.)
- Garlic powder (1.5 tsp.)
- Sliced bacon (1 lb.)
- Soft cream cheese (1 c.)

How it's made:

- Ensure that the oven can heat up to 400 degrees. Add some foil to your chosen baking sheet.
- Combine together the cream cheese, mayo, garlic powder, and cheese to make a paste.
- Slice up the peppers and fill them up with the paste you just made.
- Now use your bacon and wrap the peppers up inside of them, using a toothpick to help.
- Repeat the steps and then place the finished ones on the tray.
- Place into the oven. After twenty minutes, take out and serve warm.

Whole Food Bars

Ingredients:

- Banana (1)
- Salt
- Cinnamon (1 tsp.)
- Pumpkin puree (1 c.)
- Vanilla (1 tsp.)
- Almond butter (.5 c)
- Coconut (3 c.)

How it's made:

- Ensure that the oven heats up to 350 degrees.
- Inside your bowl, combine the vanilla, coconut, almond butter, cinnamon, and pumpkin. Make this smooth.
- Pour it out in an even layer on the baking sheet and place in the oven.
- After 25 minutes, take the dish out and cool it down a bit. Slice into squares and serve.

Goji Bars

Ingredients:

- Coconut oil (2 Tbsp.)
- Honey (2 Tbsp.)
- Cocoa powder (.5 c.)
- Hemp seeds (.5 c.)
- Dates (.5 c.)
- Shredded coconut (1 c.)
- Cashews (1 c.)
- Goji berries (.5 c.)

How it's made:

- This recipe needs the blender to start. Add in the coconut oil, coconut, honey, goji berries, cocoa powder, cashews and dates inside.
- Make this to a good mixture and pour out into a bowl with the hemp seeds.
- Spread this mixture out onto a baking sheet and place into the fridge.
- After six hours are up, take out and slice up before serving.

Cashew Butter Balls

Ingredients:

- Cashew butter (.5 c.)
- Cashews (1 c.)
- Chopped dates, pitted (1 c.)

How it's made

- Add in your cashew butter, cashews, and dates to the food processor and blend to make a nice paste.
- Using your hands, create these into balls and put onto a tray.
- Chill them for a bit before serving.

Conclusion

Thanks for making it through to the end of this book, let's hope it was informative and able to provide you with all of the tools you need to achieve your goals whatever they may be.

The next step is to get started on the sugar-free detox. This is one of the best detoxes that you can choose because it helps you to reduce the amount of sugar that you take in and, even though it only lasts for 21 days, it is long enough to help you beat your sugar addictions. Fighting off sugar can be hard, especially when hidden sugars are everywhere, but with the help of this guidebook, you will have the tools you need to get started off right.

In this guidebook, we will start off with a little information about the sugar detox before moving on to the different levels. These levels have a lot of similarities but will vary based on how closely you want to follow each one or if you would like to make some changes based on your own personal preferences. Then you will be able to find a 21-day menu plan to help you out with the sugar detox along with all the recipes that you need to make this happen. You don't need to spend hours worrying about which foods to eat and meals to prepare; all of the hard work is done for you.

After spending just three weeks on the sugar detox, you are sure to see some great results. Your energy levels will go up, your addiction to sugar will go away, and the bad health diseases you have been fighting off will finally be gone. And with the help of this guidebook, you will be able to get started with all the right tools.

Finally, if you found this book useful in any way, a review on Amazon is always appreciated!